Basic Body Detoxification and Cleansing

Anthony Parkinson, D.C.

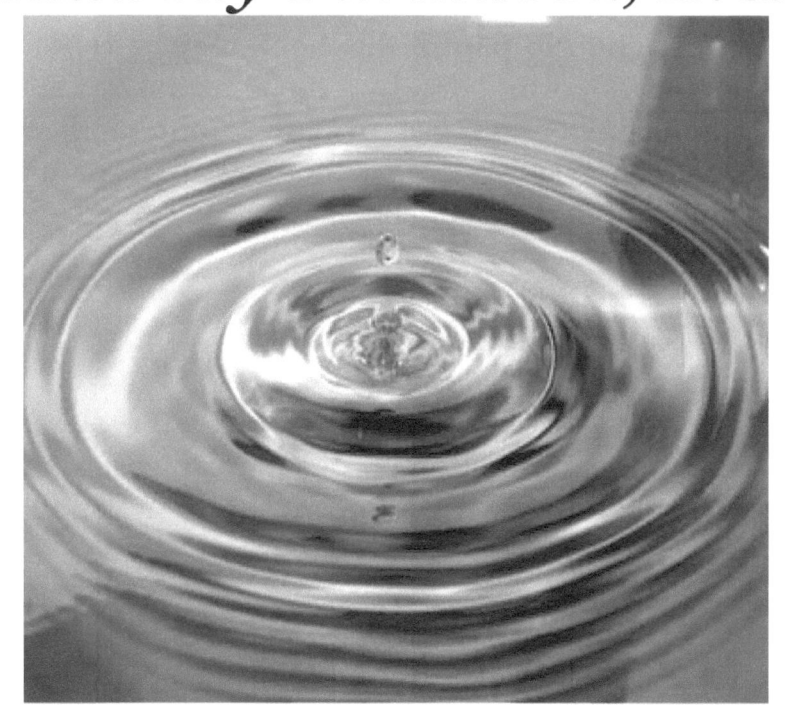

Basic Body Detoxification and Cleansing

Address:
140 Sagefield Square
Canton, MS 39046

For more information on this book, please visit the website: http//www.lulu.com/AnthonyParkinson

ISBN 978-1-4303-1418-9

Table of Contents

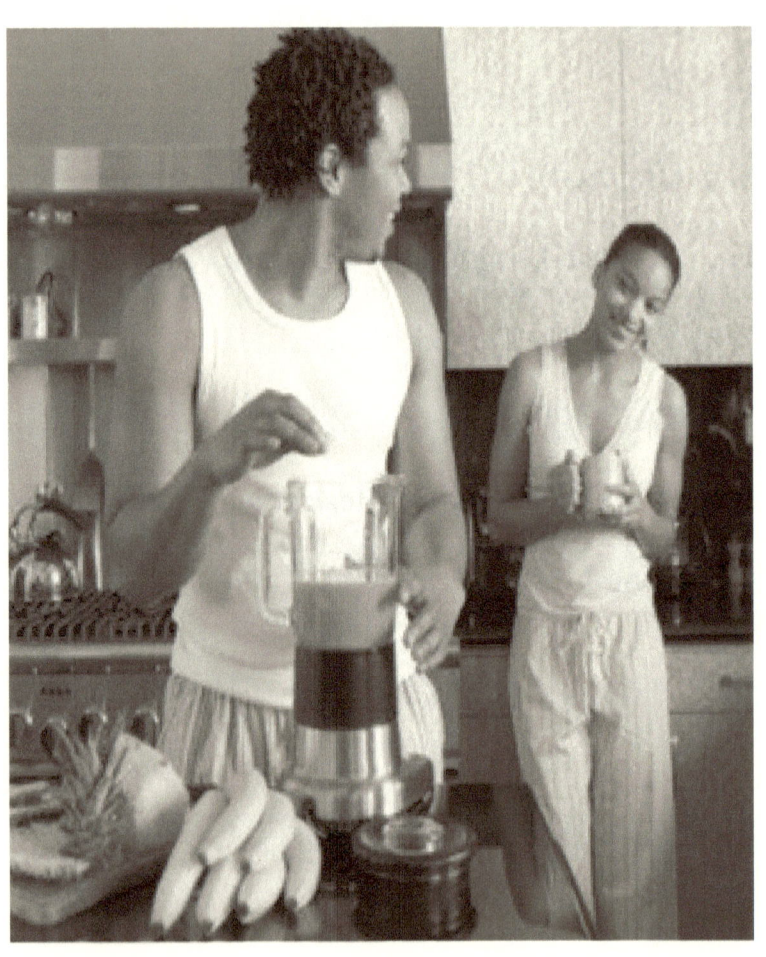

Basic Body Detoxification and Cleansing

It is somewhat difficult to separate the concepts and practices of detoxification from those of fasting. Fasting or the avoidance of solid food is one method of detoxification, probably the most effective, yet extreme, form.

There are many other ways to detoxify.

Toxicity is of much greater concern in the twentieth century than ever before. We ingest new chemicals, use more drugs of all kinds, eat more sugar and refined foods, and daily abuse ourselves with various stimulants and sedatives.

The incidence of many toxicity diseases has increased as well. Cancer and cardiovascular disease are two of the main ones. Arthritis, allergies, obesity, and many skin problems are others.

In addition, a wide range of symptoms, such as headaches, fatigue, pains, coughs, gastrointestinal problems, and problems from immune weakness, can all be related to toxicity.

Toxicity occurs on two basic levels external and internal. We can acquire toxins from our environment by breathing them, ingesting them, or through physical contact with them.

We all are exposed to toxins daily. We eat and drink them and impose them upon ourselves repeatedly and regularly. Most drugs, food additives, and allergens can create toxic elements in the body. In fact any substance can have toxicity: water, sodium, and almost all nutrients can be a problem in certain circumstances.

On the internal level, our body produces toxins through its normal everyday functions. Biochemical, cellular, and bodily activities generate substances that need to be eliminated.

When toxic substances and molecules are not eliminated, they can cause irritation or inflammation of the cells and tissues, blocking normal functions on a cellular, organ, and whole body level. Microbes of all kinds: intestinal bacteria, foreign bacteria, yeasts, and parasites produce metabolic waste products that we must handle. Our thoughts and emotions and stress itself generate increased biochemical toxicity. The proper level of elimination of these toxins is essential to health. Clearly, a normal functioning body was created to handle certain levels of toxins; the concern is with excess intake or production of toxins or a reduction in the processes of elimination.

A toxin is basically any substance that creates irritating and/or harmful effects in the body, undermining our health or stressing our biochemical or organ functions.

This may result from drugs which have side effects, or from patterns of physiology that are different from our usual functioning. Recreational drugs also usually have some harmful effects. The free radicals irritate, inflame, age, and cause degeneration of body tissues.

Negative feelings, psychic and spiritual influences, thought patterns, and negative emotions all can be toxins as well; both as stressors and by changing the normal physiology of the body and possibly producing specific symptoms.

Toxicity occurs in our body when we take in more than we can utilize and eliminate.

Homeostasis means that our body functions are in balance. This balance is disturbed when we feed ourselves more than we can utilize or partake of specific substances that are toxic.

Toxicity may depend on the dosage, frequency, or potency of the toxin. A toxin may produce an immediate or rapid onset of symptoms, as many pesticides and some drugs do; possibly, even more commonly, it may cause some long term negative effect, such as asbestos exposure leading to mesothelioma.

Of course, if our body is working well, with good immune and eliminative functions, we can handle our basic everyday exposure to toxins.

Through detoxification, we clear and filter toxins and wastes and allow our body to work on enhancing its basic functions.

Our body handles toxins by neutralizing, transforming, or eliminating them. As examples, many of the antioxidant nutrients we have discussed so much may neutralize free-radical molecules. The liver helps transform many toxic substances into harmless agents, while the blood carries wastes to the kidneys; the liver also dumps wastes through the bile into the intestines, where much waste is eliminated. We also clear toxins through sweating, from exercise or heat. Our sinuses and skin may also be accessory elimination organs whereby excess mucus or toxins can be released, as with sinus congestion or skin rashes, respectively.

Detoxification occurs on many other levels as well. Physically, this process can help clear congestions, illnesses, and disease potential. It can improve energy. Many detox processes can help rejuvenate us and prevent degeneration.

Mental detoxification is also important. Cleansing our minds of negative thought patterns is essential to health; the physical detoxification also helps this mental process. Emotionally, detoxification helps us uncover and express feelings, especially hidden frustrations, anger, resentments, or fear, and replace them with forgiveness, love, joy, and hope.

On a spiritual level, many people experience new clarity and/or an enhancement of their purpose of life during cleansing processes. A light detox over a couple of days can help us feel better, while a longer process and deeper commitment to a new way of life, such as eliminating certain abusive habits and eating a better diet, will help us really change our whole life.

Detoxification is part of a transformational medicine that instills change on many levels. Change and evolution are keys to healing.

Enhancing elimination helps one to deal with and clear problems from our past, from childhood and parental patterns to recent job or relationship stress.

When our body has eliminated much of its toxic buildup, we feel lighter and are able to really experience the moment and be open for the future.

Detoxification is a relative term. Anything that supports our elimination can be said to help us detoxify. Doing nothing more than drinking an extra quart of water a day will usually help us eliminate more toxins.

Eating more fruits and vegetables, the high water content, cleansing foods and less meat and milk products will create less congestion and more elimination.

There are many levels of the progressive detoxification diets, from these simple changes to complete fasting.

Some people go to extremes with fasting, laxatives, enemas, colonics, diuretics, and even exercise and begin to lose essential nutrients from their body.

A negative balance can be created in this manner, such as protein or vitamin and mineral deficiencies though congestion from over intake and under elimination is a more common problem in this culture.

Who Is Best Suited for Detoxification?

Almost everyone needs to detox, cleanse themselves, and rest their body functions at times. Cleansing or detoxification is one part of the trilogy of nutritional action, the others being building, or toning, and balance, or maintenance. With a regular, balanced diet, devoid of excesses, we will need less intensive detoxification.

Our body has a daily elimination cycle, mostly carried out at night and in the early morning, up until breakfast.

However, when we eat a congesting diet higher in fats, meats, dairy products, refined foods, and chemicals, detoxification becomes more necessary. Who needs to detoxify and when is based in part on individual lifestyle and needs.

More common toxicity symptoms include headache, fatigue, mucus problems, aches and pains, digestive problems, allergy symptoms, and sensitivity to environmental agents such as chemicals, perfumes, and synthetics.

People who experience these and others on the list may benefit from diet changes or avoidance of the drug or agent that may be influencing the symptom. It may be important to differentiate allergic symptoms from those of toxicity to determine the appropriate medical care.

Fasting can be extremely beneficial for people with allergies. Of course, there may be subtle characteristics of toxicity that differentiate it from other health concerns.

SIGNS AND SYMPTOMS OF TOXICITY

Headaches	Backaches	Runny nose	Fatigue
Joint pains	Itchy nose	Nervousness	Skin rashes
Cough	Frequent colds	Sleepiness	Hives
Wheezing	Irritated eyes	Insomnia	Nausea
Sore throat	Immune weakness	Dizziness	Indigestion
Tight/stiff neck	Environmental sensitivity	Mood changes	Anorexia
Angina pectoris	Sinus congestion	Anxiety	Bad breath
Circulatory deficits	Fever	Depression	Constipation
High blood fats			

Many common acute and chronic illnesses may be alleviated by a program of detoxification/cleansing, as they are basically created by short and long term congestive patterns.

People with addictions to any substance may benefit from a detox program, even if it is only the temporary avoidance of the addictive agent or agents.

Withdrawal symptoms that commonly occur with many drugs, including sugar, caffeine, and over-the-counter medications, are precipitated by detoxification.

Many of the poisons (toxins) that we ingest or make are stored in the fatty tissues.

Obesity is almost always associated with toxicity. When we lose weight, we reduce our fat and thereby our toxic load.

However, during weight loss we release more toxins, and thus need protection through greater intake of water, fiber, and the antioxidant nutrients, such as vitamins C, E, and beta-carotene, selenium, and zinc.

Problems Related to:
Congestion/Stagnation/Toxicity

Acne	Obesity	Prostate disease
Abscesses	Infections by:	Menstrual problems
Boils	*Bacteria*	Vaginitis
Eczema	*Virus*	Varicose veins
Allergies	*Fungus*	Diabetes
Arthritis	*Parasites*	Peptic ulcers
Asthma	*Worms*	Gastritis
Constipation	Uterine tumors	Pancreatitis
Colitis	Cancer	Mental illness
Hemorrhoids	Cataracts	Multiple sclerosis
Diverticulitis	Colds	Alzheimer's disease
Cirrhosis	Bronchitis	Senility
Hepatitis	Pneumonia	Parkinson's disease
Fibrocystic breast disease	Sinusitis	Drug addiction
Atherosclerosis	Emphysema	Tension headaches
Heart disease	Kidney stones	Migraine headaches
Hypertension	Kidney disease	Gallstones
Thrombophlebitis	Stroke	Gout

Of course, not all of these problems are solely problems of toxicity or completely cured by detoxification.

Most of these diseases, and the majority of those factors, have to do with abuses, especially on a nutritional level.

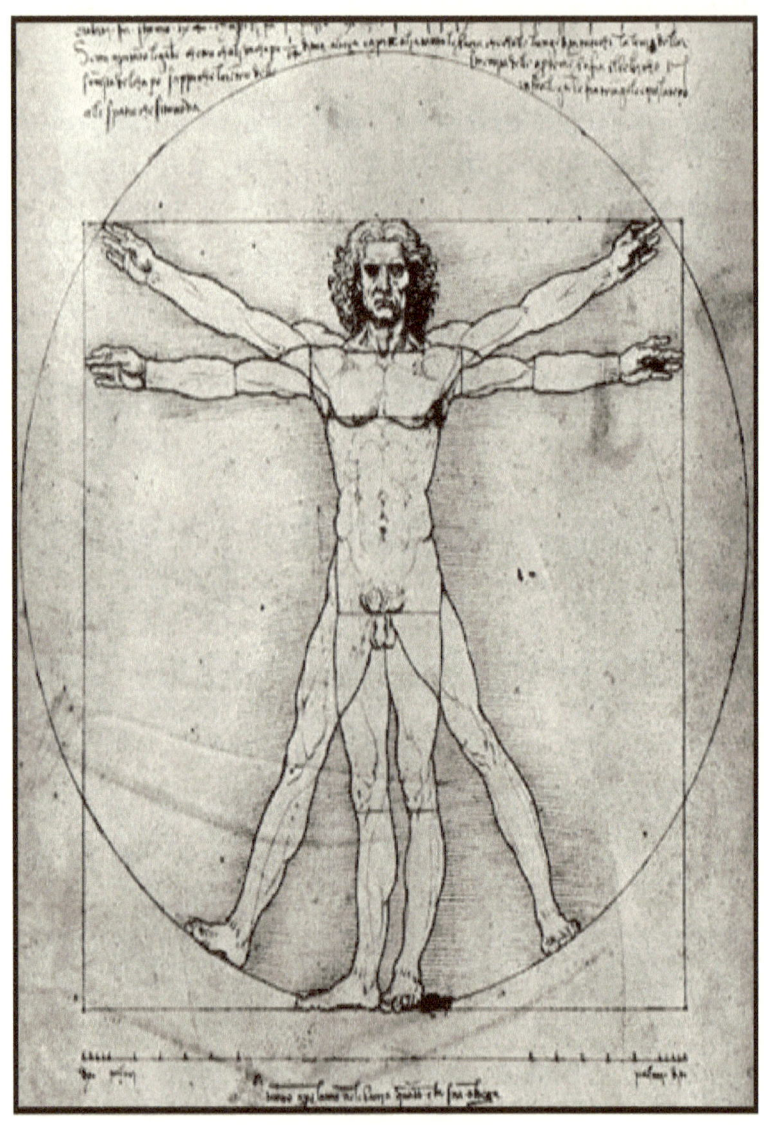

What Is Detoxification?

Detoxification is the process of clearing toxins from the body or neutralizing or transforming them, and clearing excess mucus and congestion. Many of these toxins come from our diet, drug use, and environmental exposure, both acute and chronic. Internally, fats, especially oxidized fats and cholesterol, free radicals, and other irritating molecules act as toxins.

Functionally, poor digestion, colon sluggishness and dysfunction, reduced liver function, and poor elimination through the kidneys, respiratory tract, and skin all add to increased toxicity.

Detoxification involves dietary and lifestyle changes that reduce intake of toxins and improve elimination.

Avoidance of chemicals, from food or other sources, refined food, sugar, caffeine, alcohol, tobacco, and many drugs helps minimize the toxin load.

Drinking extra water (purified) and increasing fiber by including more fruits and vegetables in the diet are steps in the detoxification process. Moving from a more to a less congesting diet will help us to move along the detox road.

Detoxification therapy, as fasting, is the oldest treatment known to humans and is a completely natural process; and in many cases, as we listen to our inner guidance as animals do, we may apply this process to many illnesses and states of health and life.

Many authorities claim the detox process helps clear wastes and old or dead cells and revitalizes the body's natural functions and healing capacities.

When Is the Best Time to Cleanse/Detoxify?

We need to incorporate nature's cycles with our own cycles. We may notice regular periods of congestion, and we may reduce or prevent these by following a more detoxifying program. Whenever we feel congested, our first step is to follow detox procedures, many of which we can fine tune in time with our experience of what works for us.

If you start to feel congestion or a cold coming on, then you can exercise and sweat, sauna or steam, drink loads of fluids, take vitamins C and A, and get a good night's sleep without eating much and almost every time you will wake up well.

Each of us has a natural cleansing time when our body wants a lighter diet, more liquids, and greater elimination than intake. This occurs daily, usually in the night until midmorning; it may occur weekly but more commonly for a few days a month. Women, in particular, are aware of this natural cleansing time with their female cycle. In fact, many women do much better premenstrually and during their periods if they follow a cleansing program of more juices, greens, lighter foods, herbs, and so on in the week before their menstruation.

The seasonal cycle is really the most important in regard to natural detoxification periods. If we can harmonize with these, we can do much to stay healthy.

The seasonal changes are the key stress times in nature and the times where we most need to lighten up our outer demands and consumptions and turn more within to listen to our inner world that mirrors the natural cycles.

Spring is the key time for detoxification; autumn is also important. At least a one to two week program is suggested at these times. In spring, we may eat more citrus fruits, fresh greens, and juices or try the Master Cleanser lemonade diet, while in autumn we may dine on other harvests, such as apples or grapes, and the many vegetables. Lots of fresh fruits and vegetables are appropriate when we are going into summer; and brown rice, vegetables, and soups may be best to simplify our diet when going into winter.

The sample yearly program provided here is designed for a basically healthy person who eats well. It would not be appropriate for those with deficiency problems such as extreme fatigue, underweight people, those who experience coldness, or those with heart weakness. There are even more contraindications for fasting, which releases more toxins than this program does.

Releasing too much toxicity can make many sick people sicker; if that happens, they will need to increase fluids and eat again until they feel better. People with cancer need to be very careful about how they detoxify.

Prior to or just after surgery is not a good time to detoxify, but after healing, say about four to six weeks later. Pregnant or lactating women should not do any heavy detoxification, though they can usually handle mild programs.

Sample Year Long Detox Programs

Spring

For 7-21 days between March 10 and April 15, use one or more of the following plans:

- Master Cleanser (lemonade diet).
- Fruits, vegetables, greens.
- Juices of fruits, vegetables, and greens.
- Herbs with any of the above.
- These plans can be alternated and even include a 3-5 day supervised water fast.
- Remember to take time (about half as long as the fast) for the transition back to the regular diet.
- Elimination and food testing can also be done at this time.

Mid-Spring

3-day cleanse at new moon time in May as a reminder and enhancer of food awareness.

Summer

One week of fruits and vegetables and/or fresh juices to usher in the warm weather sometime between June 10 and July 4.

Late Summer

3-day cleanse of fruit and vegetable juices around the new moon time in August.

Autumn

7-10 day cleanse between September 11 and October 5, such as:

- Grape fast--whole and juiced--grapes, all fresh.
- Apple and lemon juice together, diluted.
- Fresh fruits and vegetables, raw and cooked.
- Fruit and vegetable juices--fruit in the morning, vegetables in the afternoon.
- Juices plus spirulina, algae, or other green chlorophyll powders.
- Whole grains, cooked squashes and other vegetables (a lighter detox).
- Mixture of the above plans.
- Basic low-toxicity diet with herbal program.
- Colon detox with fiber (psyllium, pectin, and so on) along with enemas or colonics.
- Preparing and planning new autumn diet, enhancing positive dietary habits.

Mid-Autumn

3-day cleanse on juices or in-season produce around new moon in late October/early November.

Winter

A lighter diet in preparation for the holidays (can be done between December 10 and January 5):

- Avoidance of toxins and treats, with a very basic wholesome diet.
- One week of brown rice, cooked vegetables, miso broth, and seaweed. Ginger and cayenne pepper can be used in soups.
- Saunas or steams and massage--you deserve it!
- Hang on until spring!

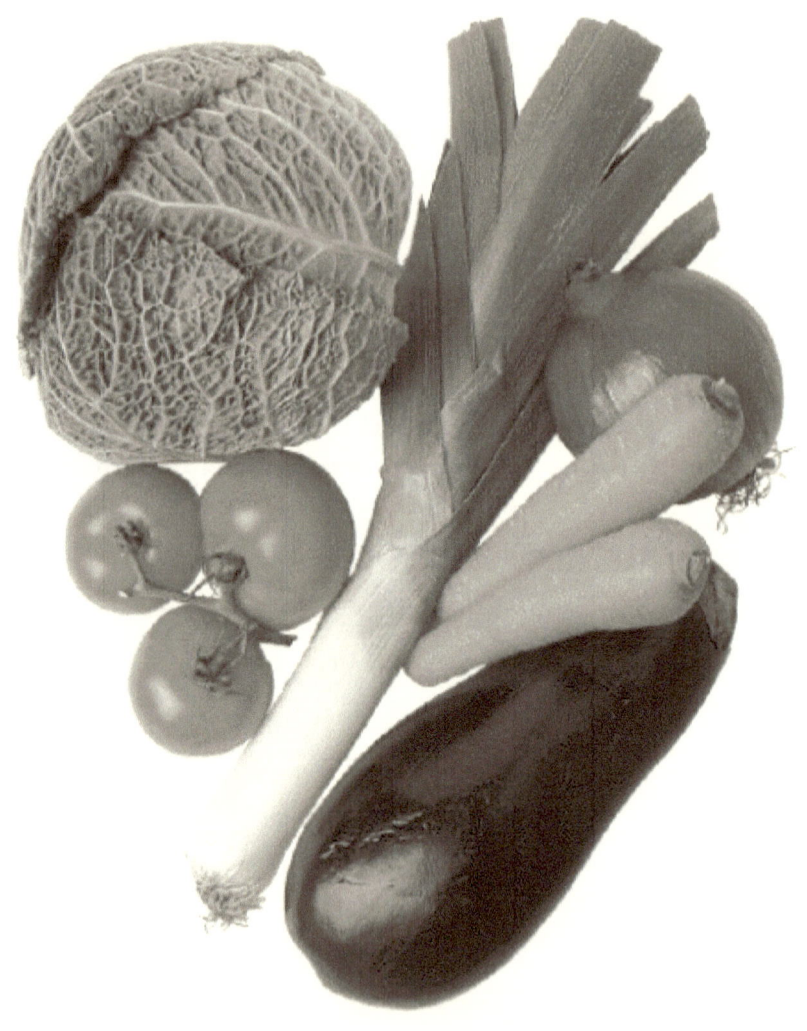

Where Can We Detoxify?

During basic, simple detox plans, most of us can maintain our normal life functions. In fact, energy, performance, and health often improve. For some though, detox may produce symptoms such as headaches, fatigue, irritability, mucous congestions, or aches and pains; any of the symptoms of toxicity may appear, though usually not.

According to naturopathic theory, any symptoms that have previously been experienced may also be experienced transiently during detox.

However, sometimes it is hard to know what is actually happening. Should we treat the problems that come up or simply watch them? Since my basic approach is to allow the body to heal itself and support the natural healing process whenever possible.

For many of us, especially the new or inexperienced, it is wise to begin any special programs, diet, or lifestyle changes with a few days at home. In time, experience will show what is best for us.

Most of us can maintain a regular work schedule during a detox or cleanse program, but it may be easier to begin a program on a Friday, as the first few days are usually the hardest.

This is because some people may be more sensitive during cleansing to their work environment or to chemical exposures, for example. Also, certain individuals may be faced with temptations or the influence of other workers or family members challenging their decisions, and for this, knowing and trusting what they are doing and having the support of a professional or group will add to their comfort and willpower.

At the end of the first day, at around dinnertime, symptoms may begin to appear, with headache and fatigue the most common, and it is good to be able to rest and spend time in familiar surroundings without a lot of outer demands. By the third day, we usually feel pretty stable and ready for work life.

However, many people like to start new programs on Monday and just know that they will do fine, using willpower and visualization to see it through.

People often feel better than ever and are able to accomplish tasks and meet challenges more easily than usual. In fact, experienced fasters may fast during busy work periods to improve their productivity.

Preparation and projection, clearing doubts and fears, and keeping a daily journal are all useful during this vital process and are crucial to any successful undertaking.

Why Detoxify?

We detoxify for many reasons, mainly to do with health, vitality, and rejuvenation; to clear symptoms, treat disease, and prevent further problems. A cleansing program is ideal for helping us to reevaluate our lives, to make changes, or to clear abuses or addictions. It takes us through our withdrawal and reduces cravings fairly rapidly, and if we are ready, we can begin a new life without the addictive habits or drugs. People cleanse because it makes them feel more productive, creative, and open to subtle and spiritual energies.

Many individuals detox or more commonly, fast on water or juices for spiritual renewal and to feel more alive, awake, and aware. It really does help move our energies from our lower centers of digestion and elimination up into our heart, mind, and consciousness centers. Detoxification can be helpful for weight loss, though it is not a primary reduction plan. However, anyone eating 4,000 calories a day of a fatty, sweet, and poorly balanced diet who begins to eat 2,000-2,500 calories of more wholesome foods will definitely experience detoxification, weight loss, and improved health. People also detoxify to rest their overloaded organs of digestion and our liver, gallbladder, and kidneys and allow them to catch up on past work. Most often our energy is increased and steadier. There are many reasons why we may want to cleanse.

Reasons for Cleansing

Prevent disease

Reduce symptoms

Treat disease

Cleanse body

Rest organs

Purification

Rejuvenation

Weight loss

Clear skin

Slow aging

Improve flexibility

Improve fertility

Enhance the senses

To be more:

Organized

Creative

Motivated

Productive

Relaxed

Energetic

Clear

Conscious

Inwardly attuned

Spiritual

Environmentally attuned

Relationship focused

How Do You Detoxify/Cleanse?

The rest of this book are general and specific diet plans, other activities, and supplements, including vitamins, minerals, amino acids, and herbs, to aid us in this healing process.

There are many levels to this part of the program. The first is to eat a nontoxic diet. If we do this regularly, we have less need for cleansing.

If we have not been eating this way, you should detoxify first and then make permanent changes.

The Nontoxic Diet

- Eat organic foods whenever possible.
- Drink filtered water.
- Rotate foods, especially common allergens, such as milk products, eggs, wheat, and yeast foods.
- Practice food combining.
- Eat a natural, seasonal cuisine.
- Include fruits, vegetables, whole grains, legumes, nuts and seeds, and, for omnivarians, some low-fat dairy products, and fresh fish (not shellfish) and organic poultry.
- Cook in iron, stainless steel, glass, or porcelain.
- Avoid or minimize red meats, cured meats, organ meats, refined foods, canned foods, sugar, salt, saturated fats, coffee, alcohol, and nicotine

Another aspect of the nontoxic diet is avoiding over-the-counter drugs, prescription, and recreational types, and substituting natural remedies, such as nutrients, herbs, and homeopathic medicines, all of which have fewer side effects. Other natural therapies, such as acupuncture, massage, and chiropractic may help in treating some problems so that we will not need drugs for them. Avoiding or minimizing exposure to chemicals at home and work is also important. This lessens our total toxic load. Substituting natural cleansers and cosmetics is helpful.

The effects of the detoxification diet may vary. Even mild changes from your current plan may produce some responses, while more dramatic dietary shifts will produce a profound cleansing. Shifting from the most congesting foods to the least; eating more fruits, vegetables, grains, nuts and legumes and less baked goods, sweets, refined foods, fried foods and fatty foods will help most of us detoxify somewhat and bring us into better balance, with more vitalized cells, organs, and body. Maintaining the same diet but adding certain supplements can also stimulate detoxification. Fiber, vitamin C, other antioxidants, chlorophyll, and glutathione, mainly as amino acid L-cysteine, will all help (see the end program following this discussion). Herbs such as garlic, red clover, Echinacea, or cayenne may also induce some detoxification. Saunas, sweats, and niacin therapy have been used to cleanse the body.

Simply increasing liquids and decreasing fats will shift the balance strongly toward improved elimination and less toxin buildup. Increased consumption of filtered water, herb teas, fruits, and vegetables and reducing fats, especially most fried food, red meats, and milk products will also help detoxification. This is a more structured, basic diet, but for most average Westerners, it will be a major shift to a cleaner diet. A vegetarian diet would also be a healthful step toward detoxification for those with some congestive problems. In general, moving from an acid generating diet to a more alkaline one, will aid the process of detoxification.

Acid forming foods, such as meats, milk products, breads and baked goods, and especially the refined sugar and carbohydrate products, will increase body acidity and lead to more mucus production and congestion to attempt to balance the body chemistry, whereas the more alkaline, wholesome vegetarian foods enhance cleansing and clarity in the body. The right balance of acid and alkaline foods for each of us is, of course, the key.

A deeper level of the detox diet is one made up exclusively of fresh fruits, fresh vegetables, either raw and cooked, and whole grains, both cooked and sprouted; however, no breads or baked goods, animal foods and dairy products, alcohol, or nuts are used. This diet keeps fiber and water intake up and helps colon detoxification.

Most people can handle this well and make the shift from their regular diet with a few days transition. Some people do well on a brown rice fast, usually for a week or two, eating three to four bowls of rice daily along with liquids such as teas.

The next level of detoxification involves a diet consisting solely of fruits and vegetables, all cleansing foods. The green vegetables, especially the chlorophyllic and high nutrient leafy greens, are very cleansing and supportive for purification of the gastrointestinal tract and the whole body.

A raw foods diet is fulfilling for many people, very high in energy and nutrition. It contains lots of sprouted greens from seeds and grains such as wheat, buckwheat, sunflower, alfalfa, and clover; sprouted beans; soaked or sprouted raw nuts; and fresh fruits and vegetables. Cooking food is not allowed with this diet; eating foods raw maintains the highest concentrations of vitamins, minerals and important enzymes, and allows them to find their way into our body and cells.

Many people feel that this is the best of diets; it can be health supportive over quite some time if it is balanced properly.

Other specialized detox diets include macrobiotics and diets that treat certain problems, such as a yeast overgrowth or allergies.

Beyond the fruit and vegetable diet are the liquid cleanses or fasts. Juices, vegetable broths, and teas can be used to purify our body and life. Miso, a paste of fermented soybean, can be used during fasting. It provides many nutrients and supports colon function and the intestinal bacteria, which help detoxification. Spirulina, an algae powder, can also be helpful to many fasters when added to juices. It provides protein to meet body needs and may aid those who experience some fatigue with fasting. Consuming fresh, diluted juices from various fruits and vegetables is safe and helpful for many conditions described in this section. Fasting experts believe that it actually works better than straight water fast, as it helps to eliminate wastes and old or dead cells while restoring and building new tissue with the easily accessible nutrients from the juices.

Water fasting is more intense, often resulting in more sickness and less energy, than fasting with juices.

The detoxification experiences can range from subtle to intense. One needs to look at a person's general health, physiological balance, energy level, and current life activities in order to set up the right program. There are a lot of possibilities. If unsure, start with your basic diet and move along the changes toward juice fasting and see how you feel. Take a couple of days for each step, and, if you feel fine, move to the next level, as described.

Levels of Dietary Detoxification

- Basic diet
- Eliminate toxins daily from more congesting to less; for example, drugs, sugar, fried foods, meats, dairy, etc. Take one to seven days.
- Fruits, vegetables, whole grains, nuts, seeds and legumes
- Raw foods
- Fruits and vegetables
- Fruit and vegetable juices
- Specific juices, Master Cleanser, apple, carrot-greens, etc.
- Water

As is true with any healing process, the plan must be followed, reevaluated, and fine- tuned to make it work to its best potential.

If people are deficient in nutrients and/or energy, they may need a higher nutrient, higher protein building diet to improve their health rather than cleanse.

Fatigue, mineral deficiencies, and low organ functions may call for this more supportive diet.

However, even in these circumstances, short cleanses, such as three days, can help eliminate old debris and prepare the body to build with healthier blocks.

Our individual detox programs can change, as our needs often vary with time. Detoxification is an individual affair, and many personal aspects are involved in devising a complete plan.

Colon cleansing is one of the most important parts of detoxification. Much toxicity comes out of the large intestine, and sluggish functioning of this organ can rapidly produce general toxicity. During a detox program, most people will work on some level with their colon. There are entire programs for colon detoxification.

A series of colonic water irrigations, best performed by a trained professional can be the focal point of a detox program, usually along with some cleansing diet and fiber supplements for toning and cleaning the colon.

During a basic dietary detox program, other, more subtle colon stimuli are usually used to enhance colon action. These may include herbal or pharmaceutical laxatives; fiber and colon detox supplements, such as psyllium seed husks alone or mixed with other agents, for example, aloe vera powder, betonite clay, and acidophilus culture. Enemas using water, herbs, or even diluted coffee (stimulates liver cleansing) may also be used.

To improve elimination through the skin, regular exercise is important to stimulate sweating.

Exercise also improves our general metabolism and helps overall with detoxification.

Regular aerobic exercise is a key to maintaining a nontoxic body, especially when we are a little abusive of various substances. On the other hand, exercise increases the production of toxins in the body, so it must be accompanied by adequate fluids, antioxidants, vitamin and mineral replenishment, and other detoxifying principles already discussed. Regular bathing is essential to cleanse the skin of the toxins it has released and to open the pores to eliminate more. Saunas and sweats are commonly used to help purify the body through enhanced skin elimination. Dry brushing the skin with an appropriate skin brush before bathing is usually suggested, especially during detox programs, to cleanse the skin of old cells and invigorate it.

Massage therapy, especially lymphatic and even deeper massage, is very useful in supporting our detox program. It stimulates elimination and body functions and promotes relaxation. Clearing tensions, worries, and other mental exhaustions also makes for a more complete detoxification.

Resting, relaxation, and recharging are important to this rejuvenation process. During detox, you may need more rest, quiet time, and sleep; although more commonly you have more energy and function better on less sleep.

Relaxation exercises help our body rebalance as our mind and attitudes stop interfering with our natural homeostasis. Practicing yoga combines quiet, yet powerful exercises with breathing awareness and regulation, allowing increased flexibility and relaxation. It may be appropriate for many to help balance more active and more contractive exercise programs, especially during detox and transition times.

Certain supplements may be used during most of these detoxification programs. However, general supplementation is less important in this detoxification program than in many of the other programs presented in this book or in the specific detox plans for drugs, alcohol, caffeine, and nicotine, when higher amounts of nutrients can ease the withdrawal transitions.

For straight juice cleansing it is recommended to use a couple of nutrients or herbs to stimulate the detox process. Potassium, extra fiber with olive oil to clear toxins from the colon, sodium alginate from seaweeds to bind heavy metals, and apple cider vinegar in water (1 tablespoon of vinegar in 8 ounces hot water) to help reduce mucus are among these.

For people beginning to detoxify with transition diets, it is often suggested to use a specialized nutrient program to help neutralize toxins and support elimination.

With weight loss, toxins stored in the fat will need to be mobilized and cleared. More water, fiber, and antioxidants will help handle this effect.

The supplement program used for general detoxification is a low dosage multiple vitamin/mineral to fulfill the basic requirements during the transitional diet. The B vitamins, particularly niacin, are important, as are minerals such as zinc, calcium, magnesium, and potassium.

The antioxidant nutrients are also important. These include basic levels of beta-carotene, vitamin A and zinc, and vitamin E and selenium, with special focus on vitamin C, probably the main detox vitamin. Some authorities believe that higher amounts of vitamin A (50,000 IUs), vitamin C (8-12 grams), and vitamin E (1,000-1,200 IUs) are helpful in detoxification.

The liver is our most important detox organ because of its many metabolic functions. Certain authorities suggest liver supportive nutrients and even a liver glandular during general detoxification.

The liver needs water and glycogen (glucose storage) as glucuronic acid for many of its detoxification functions. A higher starch or carbohydrate diet with lower levels of protein and fats is helpful.

This plan correlates with most detox diets, from juices to brown rice and vegetables. The B vitamins, especially B3 and B6, vitamins A and C, zinc, calcium, vitamin E and selenium, and L-cysteine are all also needed to support liver detoxification.

Several amino acids are helpful in detoxification, particularly the sulfur containing ones, cysteine and methionine. L-cysteine supplies sulfhydryl groups which help to prevent oxidation and to bind heavy metals, especially mercury (vitamin C and selenium also help with this). Cysteine is the precursor of glutathione, our most important detoxifier, and thus helps to counter many chemicals and carcinogens. Glutathione is part of detoxification enzymes, specifically *glutathione peroxidase* and *reductase*, which work to prevent peroxidation of lipids and to decrease many toxins, such as smoke, radiation, auto exhaust, chemicals and drugs, and many other carcinogens.

Glycine is a secondary helper. An amino acid that supports glutathione synthesis, it also decreases the toxicity of substances such as phenols or benzoic acid, the latter used as a food preservative. Other amino acids that may have mild detoxifying effects include methionine, tyrosine, and taurine.

As mentioned earlier, another detoxification supporter is fiber, as psyllium seed husks, often combined with other detox nutrients, such as pectin, aloe vera, alginates, and/or colon herbs.

This helps cleanse mucus along the small intestine, create bulk in the colon, and pull toxins from the gastrointestinal tract. When fiber is combined with one or two tablespoons of olive oil, it helps bind toxins and reduce absorption of fats as well as some basic minerals. Psyllium husks also reduce absorption of the olive oil, which is important, since it is caloric and it may have picked up fat-soluble chemicals that were released.

Take 2 grams each of psyllium and bran several times daily (with meals and at bedtime) along with one teaspoon of olive oil to help detoxify.

Acidophilus bacteria in the colon help neutralize some toxins, reduce the metabolism of other microbes, and lessen colon toxicity. Supplemental acidophilus is often added to a detox program.

Remember, water should always be used during any type of detox program to help dilute and eliminate toxin accumulations. It is likely the most important detoxifier. It helps clean us through our skin and kidneys, and it improves our sweating with exercise. Eight to ten glasses a day (depending on our size and activity level) of clean, filtered water are suggested. Some authorities suggest distilled water for use during detox programs, since, because of its lack of minerals, it will draw other particles (nutrients and toxins) to it; however, it may throw off your biochemical/electrical balance, and regular purified water is preferred.

Two or three glasses of water should be taken 30-60 minutes before each meal and even at night to help flush toxins during our body's natural elimination time.

A special elimination process has been developed and used in some clinics to help in the detoxification of chemicals, especially pesticides and even pharmaceutical drugs. This program usually involves several weeks at a center with a therapy including a high fluid and juice diet, exercise, and large amounts of niacin (vitamin B3) with sauna therapies. The saunas are extended and may last for several hours daily, with breaks to drink fluids. The idea is to cleanse the hidden chemicals from the fat through juice cleansing, weight loss, niacin therapy, exercise, and sweats.

Niacin is a vasostimulator and vasodilator, aiding circulation.

This niacin-sauna program is interesting and definitely has possibilities as an intense, medically supervised detoxification process. However, it is still experimental and does entail risks. Preliminary results are good, especially for people with symptoms caused by exposure to pesticides, such as Agent Orange, yet there are some drawbacks. Besides the cost and time required, the extreme detox can cause losses of nutrients, especially minerals, creating depletions from which it could take months to recover.

Special attention must be given to ensuring proper nutrient restoration during and after this therapy. This program, even short versions of it, can be used to help detoxify from most drugs, especially the recreational types, and daily abuses of alcohol and nicotine. Many can do a modified version with the use of a sauna, a few day's juice fast, regular exercise, and supplemental niacin, beginning at 100-200 mg. and moving up to 2-3 grams daily.

Be sure to replenish fluids and minerals. If there are medical problems, weakness or fatigue, seeks the advice and supervision of a health care provider.

Many herbs can support or even create detoxification. In fact, this area is really the strength of herbal medicine.

There are hundreds of possible herbs to be used for blood cleansing and cleaning the tissues or strengthening the function of specific organs. The following are some of the more important ones.

Cleansing Herbs

Garlic--blood cleanser, lowers blood fats, natural antibiotic

Red clover blossoms--blood cleanser, good during convalescence and healing

Echinacea--lymph cleanser, improves lymphocyte and phagocyte actions

Dandelion root--liver and blood cleanser, diuretic, filters toxins, a tonic

Chaparral--strong blood cleanser, with possibilities for use in cancer therapy

Cayenne pepper--blood purifier, increases fluid elimination and sweat

Ginger root--stimulates circulation and sweating

Licorice root--"great detoxifier," biochemical balancer, mild laxative

Yellow dock root--skin, blood, and liver cleanser, contains vitamin C and iron

Burdock root--skin and blood cleanser, diuretic and diaphoretic, improves liver function, antibacterial and antifungal properties

Sarsaparilla root--blood and lymph cleanser, contains saponins, which reduce microbes and toxins

Prickly ash bark--good for nerves and joints, anti-infectious

Oregon grape root--skin and colon cleanser, blood purifier, liver stimulant

Parsley leaf--diuretic, flushes kidneys

Goldenseal root--blood, liver, kidney, and skin cleanser, stimulates detoxification

A GENERAL CLASSIFICATION OF HERBS USEFUL IN DETOXIFICATION*

Blood Cleansers	Laxatives	Diuretics	Skin Cleansers Diaphoretics
Echinacea	Cascara sagrada	Parsley	Burdock
Red clover	Buckthorn	Yarrow	Oregon grape
Dandelion	Dandelion	Cleavers	Yellow dock
Burdock	Yellow dock	Horsetail	Goldenseal
Yellow dock	Rhubarb root	Corn silk	Boneset
Oregon grape root	Senna leaf	Uva ursi	Elder flowers
	Licorice	Juniper berries	Peppermint
			Cayenne pepper
			Ginger root

Antibiotics		Anticatarrhals**	
Garlic	Echinacea	Echinacea	Hyssop
Myrrh	Propolis	Boneset	Garlic
Prickly ash	Clove	Goldenseal	Yarrow
Wormwood	Eucalyptus	Sage	

*Not usually for fasting or juice cleansing, but mainly for dietary detoxification--using herbs alone may be the most productive in some detoxification programs. Consult a naturopathically oriented doctor.

**anti-catarrhals help eliminate mucus

SAMPLE DETOX FORMULA

Echinacea   *Garlic*

Goldenseal root   *Parsley leaf*

Yellow dock root   *Licorice root*

Cayenne pepper

Obtain powders (or ground herb), equal amounts.

www.ingramcontent.com/pod-product-compliance
Lightning Source LLC
Chambersburg PA
CBHW021548290526
45784CB00016B/2647